Make Fitness a Priority Workbook

A Six-Week Course to Get out of Your Own Way

CHAD AUSTIN

Disclaimer:

Although the author and publisher have made every effort to ensure that the information in this book was correct at press time, the author and publisher do not assume and hereby disclaim any liability to any party for any loss, damage, or disruption caused by errors or omissions, whether such errors or omissions result from negligence, accident, or any other cause.

This book is not intended as a substitute for the medical advice of physicians. The reader should regularly consult a physician in matters relating to his/her health and particularly with respect to any symptoms that may require diagnosis or medical attention.

The information in this book is meant to supplement, not replace, proper fitness training. Like any sport involving speed, equipment, balance and environmental factors, fitness training poses some inherent risk. The author and publisher advise readers to take full responsibility for their safety and know their limits. Before practicing the skills or methods described in this book, be sure that your equipment is well maintained, and do not take risks beyond your level of experience, aptitude, training, and comfort level.

Contents

Introduction

What are your top priorities in life? I've done a lot of research on this question, so I can tell you that the top answers people usually give are family and career. The answer that most people wouldn't even think about giving is fitness. This surprising statistic is what inspired me to write my best-selling book, *Make Fitness a Priority: How to Win the Fight Against Your Excuses.*

In our minds, fitness is always something that we plan to get to later because we think we are too busy now. We all have obstacles and challenges in our lives that we can use as excuses to put fitness off until later.

Obstacles like:

- I'm too busy. I don't have any time to work out.

- I'm too tired. I don't have any energy left to work out.

- I travel all the time for work. I never know where I'm going or when I'm going. That makes it impossible for me to get into a consistent routine.

- I have kids at home I need to be there for. My kids have activities going on every other night of the week, and I need to be there to support them.

- I don't have a gym nearby to go to.

- Even if I did have a gym nearby to go to, I wouldn't have any idea what to do when I walked in the door.

Do any of those statements sound familiar? Have you used any of them? We use these obstacles as validation to ourselves that it is just not in the cards for us to get in shape right now. Our fitness is always the thing we put off until later . . . you know, when we have more time. The problem with that way of thinking is that magical day we are waiting for when all of sudden we won't be busy anymore and we will have tons of free time—that day will never come. It does not exist. That is the realization you need to make right now. I really hate to be the one to break it to you, but there will never be a shortage of excuses. There will always be excuses you can use to skip your workout and validate going through the drive-through.

Let's say instead of asking you what are your top priorities in life, I asked you what are some things you can do to improve your quality of life. For that question, I am sure that exercising and eating healthy would be two of the top answers. In this six-week workbook, my goal is not to convince you that exercising and eating right is important. You already understand the value of those things. My goal is to help you realize that even though you are busy and you have obstacles and challenges that you face regularly, you can still make fitness a priority in your life too. If you decide to do that, your quality of life will be better.

After completing this six-week program, you will:

1. Realize that every excuse is just an obstacle you have not overcome yet.

2. Learn how to set yourself up for success at the beginning of every week, and put a stop to your excuses before they show up.

3. Learn how to evaluate yourself at the end of every week and become a problem solver for every challenging obstacle you face.

4. Be able to use your WHY FUEL to help you get long-term success and stop starting over.

5. Understand that failing is inevitable, but it doesn't end your fitness journey.

6. Learn that anyone, no matter what obstacles they face, can make fitness a priority in their lives, and if you choose to do it, your life will be better.

Change Your Mindset with the Fit List Test

I'm too busy. . . I'm too tired. . . I'm too bored. . . Are you having a tough time getting past your excuses? The Fit List Test will help you quickly change your mindset from "I'm too busy; I can't do this right now" to "I can do this right now, and if I do it will make my life better."

Step 1:

In the table below you will make a list of your fitness heroes. Your fitness heroes are the people who, in your mind, always make fitness a priority in their lives. Despite whatever obstacles or challenges they may regularly face, they always find a way to get their workouts in and stick to a healthy eating routine.

Your Fitness Heroes

Step 2:

In the following table, make a list of all of the obstacles that your fitness heroes overcome in order to make fitness a priority. For example: they have a very busy schedule, they have a stressful job, they have to travel a lot for work, they have kids at home, their kids are always involved in activities they need to be at, they are a single parent, they don't have a gym close by to go to, they have an illness/disability . . . etc.

Obstacles Your Fitness Heroes Face and Overcome	
Your Fitness Heroes	Your Hero's Obstacles
	1. 2. 3.
	1. 2. 3.
	1. 2. 3.
	1. 2. 3.
	1. 2. 3.

Step 3:

In the table below, make a list of all of the obstacles that are often in your way and make it difficult to make fitness a priority in your life.

Obstacles You Have in Your Way

Step 4:

Take some time to compare the lists you made in steps 2 and 3. Who faces the most obstacles, you or your fitness heroes? Whose obstacles are bigger?

Step 5:

The lesson that you learn from taking this test is that everyone has to face obstacles when making fitness a priority. There will also always be obstacles that you have to overcome. The obstacles will change from time to time, but there will always be obstacles in the way. The reason that your heroes are able to always make fitness a priority in their lives, no matter what challenges are in their way, is that they have made it very important to them. They have a very strong reason WHY they make fitness a top priority in their lives, and that gives them the strength to overcome any obstacle they face. You can do that too! We will dig deeper into what your WHY is in Week 1, but take some time to think about this now. Why is making fitness a priority important to you?

Week 1
The Plan of Attack

Making fitness a priority in your life is not easy. That is one thing my clients will never hear me say. Everyone has their own set of challenges that they must overcome. Sometimes it is a real fight, but it is a fight that anyone can win. The reward for accepting this challenge is greatly improving your quality of life.

When it comes to your health and fitness regimen, success begins the same way it does with your job, with your family, and with every other priority in your life. You must make a plan. You can start with the best intentions in the world, but if you don't have a plan, you may as well plan to fail. At my personal training studio, Priority Fitness, in Overland Park, Kansas, I help my clients reach their goals with a Mindset-Nutrition-Training approach.

Mindset:

The first step to making fitness a priority is changing your mindset. In order to get long-term success, you must begin this program with no end in mind. Just because this is a six-week workbook does not mean that your fitness journey will end after Week 6. My goal with this workbook is to help you make lifestyle changes and build habits that you can continue using long after you finish this book. You must think of this as the first six weeks of fitness being a priority in your life.

Nutrition:

Every successful fitness program must start with good nutrition. It's simple . . . you can't out-train a bad diet. No matter what your goals are, if you are not fueling your body the right way, you will not get the results you want.

Training:

Just like having the right mindset and eating healthy, the training part of fitness comes with no shortage of challenges. The lessons in this workbook are designed to help you find a program that works best for you and teach you how to get the most out of it.

We will begin each week of this program with new action steps in each of these categories.

Mindset: What, Why & How

Before we get any further into this program, we need to take time to set some goals. To set powerful goals, you have to ask yourself three questions:

1. What do you want to accomplish?

2. Why is this important to you?

3. How do you plan to do it?

If you just answer question 1, then you're not really setting a goal, you are actually making a wish. If you don't answer questions 2 and 3, then not only will you not take enough action, but when the going gets tough, you will not have enough motivation to keep going. To get the best results, you need to answer all three of these questions in great detail.

Short-term goals are important to get us started sometimes, but if you want to get long-term success, you must dig a little deeper. Ask yourself WHY these goals are important to you. You must figure out what your deeper motivation is.

Dig Deeper to Learn: What, Why & How

Good goals fuel motivation for long-term success! Try this formula to make your fitness goals.

The **WHAT** is easy. Just write down what you want. Be specific.

After you have everything written down comes the most important part. Ask yourself, **WHY** you want this. Be very specific. Your WHY will be the number one driving force behind your action plan. You can and will do anything with a big enough WHY. Would you run across a busy freeway for a briefcase full of pennies? What if it had a million dollars in it? What if it was to rescue your child? See . . . WHY is everything.

Once you have your WHY as fuel, you are ready to take action. Make a game plan of **HOW** you are going to accomplish your goal, and then keep yourself accountable to your plan.

Take some time to right now to make three fitness goals that fuel you for long-term success.

<u>Goal 1:</u>

What-_____

_____

_____

Why-_____

_____

_____

How-_____

_____

_____

<u>Goal 2:</u>

What-_____

_____

_____

Why-_____

_____

_____

How-_____

_____

_____

<u>Goal 3:</u>

What-_____

_____

_____

Why-_____

_____

_____

How-_____

_____

_____

Nutrition: Throw Out the Temptation

It is now time to talk about the base of the pyramid, which is nutrition. As I said earlier, no matter what your fitness goals are, accomplishing them starts with nutrition. No matter how hard you work, you simply can't out-train a bad diet. I approach nutrition with my clients the same way I approach all other aspects of fitness.

It's widely quoted that 95 percent of people regain lost weight. I bet you have heard a statistic similar to that before, and it can make you wonder why you should even bother. Before you turn your treadmill into a coat rack or a sanctuary for unfolded laundry, stop and think about why so many people fail. It has nothing to do with their goals being set too high. They are simply starting with the wrong mindset.

People fail to achieve long-term results because they have the "diet" mentality. For most people, the word diet refers to a period of time when they will have to practice superhuman willpower to resist foods they love. It will be torture, but at the end they will get to reward themselves with junk food again.

Maybe fewer people would get sucked into the diet craze if they thought of the word the same way a personal trainer does. To me, diet just means temporary results. There will always be plenty of fad diets to choose from, but none of them will ever get you long-term results. The diet mindset will always backfire because you can't sustain that way of eating forever.

I want my clients make changes that help them achieve long-term success and that they can follow for the rest of their lives. By making little changes to their eating habits, my clients have found they get more out of their workouts and have less stress, increased energy, improved moods, and get much better results. I have learned over the years that learning about nutrition can be very overwhelming. There is just so much to learn, and always something you could be doing better.

It has been my experience that when you try to change too much at once, you usually end up changing nothing at all. For that reason, I always teach my nutritional guidelines in easy-to-follow steps. Over the next few chapters, you will learn about the healthy habits that I believe everyone should follow.

Step 1: Surround yourself with healthier choices.

One of the first assignments I give every new client is to set themselves up for success at home. When we first get started, most of us are set up to fail. We are set up to fail because of all of the unhealthy choices that surround us. We have to fix this from the beginning.

Your job is to look in your refrigerator, search through your cabinets, and get rid of all the unhealthy choices that you really don't need. We make all kinds of excuses as to why we have these unhealthy items in the house, but the bottom line is we don't need them. You say you don't eat them. Are you in denial? Regardless of the reason you have them, why surround yourself with temptation?

Don't get me wrong, a cheat meal is ok from time to time and, in my opinion, can be beneficial to long-term success. Having these unhealthy choices at such easy access is just setting yourself up to fail right off the bat. Get started on the right foot. Throw out all the temptation. Get rid of all the unhealthy choices and then go get groceries and surround yourself with healthier snack and meal options.

I know I haven't talked about what healthier choices are yet, but trust me—if you know what the unhealthy choices are, then you know enough to make better choices. Fruits and vegetables are better choices than many things you may be used to having around as snacks. In the next few chapters, you will learn more tips that will help you when grocery shopping.

Action Step:

Do this step on your own right now. Look through your refrigerator and kitchen cabinets. Throw out the temptation and then set yourself up to succeed.

Training: Your Workout Plan

When it comes to working out, if you want to be successful, you must have a plan. You can have great intentions on exercising, but without a plan you might as well plan to fail. You need to know ahead of time what you are going to do for your workout, where you are going to do it, and when you are going to do it. This looks a little different for everyone, and it is important to create a plan that best fits you.

Let's Get Started

Resistance training and cardio training are both important. Think of resistance training as strength training for your muscles, and cardio training as strength training for your heart.

Some benefits of Strength Training and Cardio Training include:

Increased Strength	Increased Energy	Increased Flexibility
Better Mood	More Self-Confidence	Reduced Stress
Reduced Anxiety	Weight Loss	Weight Management
Decreased Risk of Illness		

Which of these health benefits are most important to you?

_____

_____

_____

I recommend two or three total-body resistance training workouts each week, and two or three cardio workouts per week (30–45 minutes). To help create your game plan, answer the following questions:

Where do you plan to work out?

Home   Gym   Other

How much time do you have to work out?

15–30 minutes   45 minutes or more

What days/times during the week are best for you to work out?

_____

_____

_____

What exercise experience do you have?

Beginner   Moderate   Advanced

Is this overwhelming? Want your workouts created for you?

You can work out with me online with my Make Fitness a Priority Training Program.

Program includes:

- 3 total-body resistance training workouts per week
- A very user-friendly app
- Videos demonstrating every exercise
- 2 cardio workouts (Many different cardio choices to help you find something you like.)
- Move your workouts around in your schedule to avoid conflicts
- Check in for your workouts and log your stats for every workout
- Home version and a gym version

This 4-week program is usually $79.99, but you can get it for $49.99*

Purchase here: https://overlandparkfitness.com/product/make-fitness-a-priority-online-training-program/

*At checkout, enter Promo Code: **MFAPworkbook**

Want to create your own program instead?

Use your answers to the questions above and follow the steps below to fill out the workout schedule on the next page.

1. Where you will do your workouts: Home or Gym.
2. For each week, write in the days you plan to do your resistance training workouts.
3. By each scheduled resistance training workout, include where you will be doing it (home or gym) and what time you plan to do it (Ex: 5 a.m. before work, or 5 p.m. after work).
4. Repeat steps 2 and 3 to schedule your cardio workouts.

Note: You can do a resistance training workout and a cardio training workout on the same day if needed.

Workout Plan							
	Sunday	Monday	Tuesday	Wednes-day	Thursday	Friday	Saturday
Week 1							
Resistance Training							
Cardio Training							
Week 2							
Resistance Training							
Cardio Training							
Week 3							
Resistance Training							
Cardio Training							
Week 4							
Resistance Training							
Cardio Training							
Week 5							
Resistance Training							
Cardio Training							

Want more direction? Get a program made for you here:

https://overlandparkfitness.com/product/make-fitness-a-priority-online-training-program/

At checkout, use promo code: **MFAPworkbook**

$30 savings with promo code!

Now you have a plan. All you have to do is stick to it!

Weekly Fitness Evaluation Form

Now, it is time to give yourself a grade for the week. By doing this weekly self-evaluation and asking yourself the questions on this sheet, you will learn how to keep yourself accountable to your fitness plan. Every week you will learn more from doing this evaluation, and before long your fitness plan will become a top priority in your life.

Here is how this works: Answer the questions below, and then grade yourself for the week. If you give yourself an A+, awesome! All you have to do is just keep it up. If you don't give yourself an A+, ask yourself what went wrong. What obstacles got in your way? How can you overcome these obstacles in the future? These questions will help you when setting yourself up for next week's success.

First, let's start with what you did well . . .

Name three things you are proud of after this week:

1._____

2._____

3._____

Mindset

How was your energy this week? If it was low, did you get enough sleep? Did you drink enough water? What other factors could've affected your energy?

_____

_____

_____

How did you feel during your workouts this week? (Ex: strong or weak, athletic or uncoordinated, tired or energetic)

_____

_____

_____

How was your motivation this week? Was it easy to get your workouts in or challenging? Was it easy to stick to the healthy guidelines or challenging?

_____

_____

_____

What grade do you give your mindset for this week? ___

Nutrition

Did you throw out the temptations and replace them with healthier options?

_____

_____

_____

Did you follow a meal plan? Did you get all your meals in? Did you drink enough water?

_____

_____

_____

Did you have any treats or cheats? If yes, what were your cheat meals? Were they intentional or unplanned?

_____

_____

_____

What grade do you give your nutrition this week? ___

Training

Did you get all of your workouts in this week (resistance training and cardio training)? If your answer is no, which workouts did you miss/skip? Why didn't you get them in?

_____

_____

_____

Did you need to make modifications to any exercises this week? If yes, which exercises, and why/how did you modify them?

_____

_____

_____

What grade do you give your workouts this week? ___

You will use your answers to the questions in this evaluation in the next section, "Set Yourself Up for Success."

Set Yourself Up for Success
in Week 2

Now, it's time to set yourself up for success for the upcoming week. Your fitness goals are no different than anything else you want to accomplish in life. If you don't have a plan, then you might as well plan to fail. The action steps in this form are designed to help you reach your goals in the week ahead.

The first thing we're going to do is overcome the biggest excuse that we always make: "I don't have time." We love this excuse, and it is the easiest one to use.

Make Time

We are going to overcome this excuse right now by making time. The way you make time is scheduling your workouts.

Step 1: Go to your online training program and click on your calendar. I have scheduled your workouts out for the week, but you have the ability to drag and move them to whatever day you'd like. (Not doing one of my online training programs? No problem. You can use your phone calendar or your desk calendar, and just move your workouts around any conflicts.)

Step 2: Identify any conflicts that could affect your workouts getting completed. Look at your work schedule this week. Do you have to travel this week? Are there any meetings or events you need to be at that could be overlapping a scheduled workout? Now look at your family calendar. What family stuff is going on this week? Do you have a family event or activity going on this week? Do you have a date with a significant other? Do your kids have activities or events this week? What conflicts present themselves?

Step 3: Drag and move your workouts around any conflicts that you face this week. (It is ok to do resistance training workouts on consecutive days if you have to in order to get them in. Ideally, you want to have a rest day between them when possible. It is also ok to do a resistance training workout and a cardio workout on the same day.)

Step 4: Plan out what time of day you will be doing each workout. (In the morning before work, during lunch, after work, on your day off. . .)

Plan Out Your Meals

What I have found to be the most successful way of keeping myself honest to a healthy eating plan throughout the week is meal prepping at the beginning of the week. You must plan out what you're going to eat throughout the week, and prepare it before the week starts. This helps set you up for success. So for example, if I know that every day for breakfast (or for one of my early morning snacks) I'm going to have two hard-boiled eggs and a banana, then on Sunday I'll purchase it, prepare it, and get it ready for the entire week. Meal prepping like this at the beginning of the week, for as many meals and snacks as you can, will help you succeed.

Step 1: In the first chart below, write out everything you plan to eat for your meals and snacks for the upcoming week. (If you are like me and eat the same thing for breakfast every day and repeat snacks often, this will not take very long.) As you fill this out for the week, be sure to write down any planned dinners out, work-related lunches or other meals, events, happy hours, etc.

Step 2: Look over the meals and snacks you planned out for the week and use the second chart to create your grocery list.

Step 3: Get your groceries for the week.

Step 4: Cook/prepare all of your meals for the week.

Meals / Snacks					
	Breakfast	AM Snack (optional)	Lunch	PM Snack (optional)	Dinner
Monday					
Tuesday					
Wednesday					
Thursday					
Friday					
Saturday					
Sunday					

Grocery List
1.
2.
3.
4.
5.
6.
7.
8.
9.
10.

Week 2
You Have the Power to Change Your Story

Usually when someone begins a new training program, they are fueled by short-term motivation. There is something coming up in the near future that they want fast results for. Perhaps it is something like a vacation, a wedding, a reunion, swimsuit season, etc. Motivation is awesome, and there is nothing wrong with using something fast-approaching to spark some fire in you to get started. The problem is that if you don't eventually look past the event and take some time to dig deeper into WHY you want the results you're chasing, all the results you get will just be temporary. Why? Because all the motivation will be gone once the event is over.

Think about all of the programs and challenges you have taken on in your past. You worked hard, and you got great results. You earned those results, but they eventually went away. They became only temporary results because you never looked past the event you were training hard for. Have you been through this pattern before? Most of us have. If you are tired of always starting over, you need to realize that you can change your story.

You must not go into this six-week program with the mindset that it is only six weeks long. Instead, have the mindset that this is just the first six weeks and have no end in mind. Instead of starting over again in the future, make fitness a priority for the rest of your life starting today.

Action Steps:

Before you start Week 2 of this program, take a second to remind yourself of your WHY. Use that WHY FUEL to motivate you this week.

Mindset: Overcoming the "I'm Too Bored" Obstacle

One problem that many of us suffer from that can lead to a big roadblock is getting bored with our workout program. This happens to us because we are creatures of habit. We fall in love with a workout routine, and then we never ever change it.

When we do the same thing for too long, not only does the inevitable happen and we eventually get insanely bored, but our bodies actually adapt to what we are doing. Once our bodies adapt to our workout routine, we stop getting results. What happens when we stop getting results? We stop having motivation to do the work in the first place.

An easy solution to overcoming the "I'm too bored" obstacle is something I learned many years ago before I became a personal trainer. I was a PE teacher for three years before I became a personal trainer. When I was student-teaching, I was having trouble coming up with a lesson plan for a second grade class I was teaching. I was trying to come up with a new tag game, and I was all out of ideas. My cooperating teacher at the time gave me a tip that I have used throughout my whole career as a personal trainer. She said, "If you just change one little thing, those kids will think it is a completely different game." I've learned that our bodies and minds act the exact same way when it comes to our exercises and workouts. If we just change a few little things in our workouts, our bodies will think it is completely different. We won't get bored, and we will keep getting results.

There are so many variables that you can change to make your workouts a little different.

First, you can just change the equipment in your workouts. Instead of using dumbbells, you can use barbells. Instead of using cables, you can use resistance bands. Instead of using machines, you can utilize bodyweight exercises.

You can change the sets, reps, and/or tempo. Instead of making one circuit of six exercises you could do two circuits of three exercises. Instead of doing higher reps of 12–15 per exercise you could do more sets of lower reps of 8–10 reps per exercise. Instead of doing your reps at your normal speed, you could speed the pace up to be more explosive, or slow it down and focus more on form.

You could change your schedule or frequency of workouts. Instead of training for an hour three days per week, you could train for forty-five minutes four days per week. You could take away a resistance training day, and elect to do a bootcamp class or cardio class instead.

The options for change are endless, and remember that it doesn't have to be a big change. Even a small change can keep you from falling into the "this is boring" trap.

Action Steps: Keep these tips in mind as you start getting into a workout routine. If you start getting bored, use them as a guide to change things up.

Nutrition: Healthy Eating Guidelines
Part 1

As a personal trainer, I have learned a lot about nutrition over the years in order to help my clients succeed. Every fitness certification I have has come with more education in nutrition, but like most personal trainers, I am not a licensed dietician or a nutritionist. I have, however, gained a wealth of knowledge about healthy eating over the years through education and experience. When it comes to improving your nutrition habits, there are always more changes you can make to improve your health. One thing I know for sure is that when someone tries to change too many things at once in their life, they end up changing nothing. For that reason, I have my clients only focus on making two or three changes at a time. Once your healthy changes become habits, then you can add more.

Over the next few weeks, I will be sharing two or three healthy eating guidelines each week for you to incorporate into your life. For this week we will introduce three.

1. Don't Skip Breakfast

I would say half of the people I meet tell me they skip breakfast most mornings. I'm sure you have heard the phrase "breakfast is the most important meal of the day." Well, it is. It gets your metabolism going and gives your brain and body the energy it desperately needs after fasting all night. It's called "breakfast" because it breaks our fast.

For most people, the time they spend in bed is the longest period they go without food. When you get up in the morning, it may be eight to twelve hours since you last ate, and now your blood sugar level is at rock bottom. In order for your brain to function properly, it needs a constant supply of sugar, which is why starting your day with a good breakfast is so important. You need fuel to function. Let's say you had dinner at 7 p.m. the night before. Then, when you leave for work at 7 a.m., you forget to eat breakfast. That is twelve hours without putting gas in the tank. If you don't eat your first meal until lunch time, that is probably another five hours. That's seventeen hours without refueling.

No wonder we are so tired all the time. We spend most of the day running on fumes. Imagine how much more energy you would have, and how much more productive you would probably be, if you refueled before leaving for work.

2. Eat Three Meals A Day (Breakfast, Lunch & Dinner)

While breakfast is thought by many to be the most important meal of the day, it will not get you through the entire day all by itself. Think of your body as a car. For it to run at its best, it needs to be taken care of and refueled regularly. Your body is the same way. If you do not refuel during the day, you will be running on fumes by the early afternoon. For best results, begin eating breakfast, lunch, and dinner every day.

3. Stay Hydrated

Water is our bodies' most important nutrient, and many of us don't get enough of it. It is crazy how many annoying issues such as headaches, dizziness, fatigue, and lack of strength can simply be the result of being dehydrated. The human body is predominantly water and functions best when it is properly hydrated. You should drink half your body weight in ounces every day. I know half your body weight may seem like a lot, but this little adjustment will do wonders. Along with these daily requirements for water, you must also replace the water you lose during your workouts, from sweating ,and from any diuretics (coffee, alcohol, etc.) you drink during the day.

Tip: Start your day by drinking a big glass of cold water. It's an easy habit to get into and will give your metabolism a jumpstart in the morning. Put a glass of water next to your alarm clock before you go to sleep, then it will be waiting for you first thing in the morning.

Action Steps:

How will you incorporate these guidelines this week?

_____

_____

_____

How can you ensure success in adding these new healthy habits?

_____

_____

_____

Training: Modifications Will Help You Progress

As you start going through your workouts, keep in mind that every exercise can be made easier or it can be made harder. If an exercise is a little bit too hard, don't skip it, just modify it to the current fitness level you are now. For example, if a sit-up is just a little bit too hard—say it hurts your back or you can't quite get the full range of motion—just make it a crunch. If a push-up is too hard for you to do with good form, there are many ways you can modify it. You can do it on your knees, or you can move your hands to a bench or a bar so it's higher. If jumping or hopping is a little bit too hard starting out, then just take the impact away and keep it as a regular squat or a lunge. Any exercise can be modified. See the chart below.

Don't let it frustrate you if you have to modify an exercise. Modifications will actually help make you better. If an exercise is too hard and you need to modify it, it doesn't mean that you can't do it, it simply means you can't do it yet. If you keep making modifications as you go through the workouts, you'll notice that you'll improve so much faster that way.

When exercises are a little too hard, you just have to regress them a little to finish your workout. At the same time, as you get consistent with your workout routine, you will notice some exercises becoming too easy. These exercises you can progress. See chart for examples.

Modifications are easy to make during your workouts. Just think, "How can I make this just a little easier (or harder)?" Modify things as needed, but don't skip anything. If you need any help with modifications as you go through your workouts, just reach out to me, and I'll help walk you through it.

Modifications Chart:

Regressions		Exercise	Progressions	
Crunch	Long Lever Crunch	Sit-up	Sit-up with weight	Sit-up to Balance Hold
Low Plank on Bench	High Plank (on Hands)	Low Plank (on elbows)	Low Plank on BOSU	Low Plank with Feet on BOSU
Push-up from Knees	Push-up on Bench	Push-up	Push-up on BOSU	Push-up with Feet on BOSU
Stability Ball Squat	Bodyweight Box Squat	Bodyweight Squat	DB Squat	DB Squat Jump
Bodyweight Row	Pull-up on Machine (or with Band Assistance)	Pull-up	Pull-up with Knee Raises	L-position Pull-up

When it comes to making modifications to progress or regress an exercise, don't overthink it. This chart is just a guide and isn't based on anything scientific. Modifications look different for everybody, and what is a good modification for one person might not be a good modification for you. There is no wrong answer. The goal is always just to get the most out of your workout. The only wrong answer is to skip an exercise.

Action Step:

What are a few exercises that you regularly modify (make harder or easier)?

_____

_____

_____

How do you modify them?

_____

_____

_____

Weekly Fitness Evaluation Form

Now, it is time to give yourself a grade for the week. By doing this weekly self-evaluation and asking yourself the questions on this sheet, you will learn how to keep yourself accountable to your fitness plan. Every week you will learn more from doing this evaluation, and before long your fitness plan will become a top priority in your life.

Here is how this works: Answer the questions below, and then grade yourself for the week. If you give yourself an A+, awesome! All you have to do is just keep it up. If you don't give yourself an A+, ask yourself what went wrong. What obstacles got in your way? How can you overcome these obstacles in the future? These questions will help you when setting yourself up for next week's success.

First, let's start with what you did well . . .

Name three things you are proud of after this week:

1._____

2._____

3._____

Mindset

How was your energy this week? If it was low, did you get enough sleep? Did you drink enough water? What other factors could've affected your energy?

_____

_____

_____

How did you feel during your workouts this week? (Ex: strong or weak, athletic or uncoordinated, tired or energetic)

_____

_____

_____

How was your motivation this week? Was it easy to get your workouts in or challenging? Was it easy to stick to the healthy guidelines or challenging?

_____

_____

What grade do you give your mindset for this week? ___

Nutrition

Did you throw out the temptations and replace them with healthier options?

_____

_____

_____

Did you follow a meal plan? Did you get all your meals in? Did you drink enough water?

_____

_____

_____

Did you have any treats or cheats? If yes, what were your cheat meals? Were they intentional or unplanned?

_____

_____

_____

What grade do you give your nutrition this week? ___

Training

Did you get all of your workouts in this week (resistance training and cardio training)? If your answer is no, which workouts did you miss/skip? Why didn't you get them in?

_____

_____

_____

Did you need to make modifications to any exercises this week? If yes, which exercises, and why/how did you modify them?

_____

_____

_____

What grade do you give your workouts this week? ___

You will use your answers to the questions in this evaluation in the next section, "Set Yourself Up for Success."

Set Yourself Up for Success
in Week 3

Now, it's time to set yourself up for success for the upcoming week. Your fitness goals are no different than anything else you want to accomplish in life. If you don't have a plan, then you might as well plan to fail. The action steps in this form are designed to help you reach your goals in the week ahead.

The first thing we're going to do is overcome the biggest excuse that we always make: "I don't have time." We love this excuse, and it is the easiest one to use.

Make Time

We are going to overcome this excuse right now by making time. The way you make time is scheduling your workouts.

Step 1: Go to your online training program and click on your calendar. I have scheduled your workouts out for the week, but you have the ability to drag and move them to whatever day you'd like. (Not doing one of my online training programs? No problem. You can use your phone calendar or your desk calendar, and just move your workouts around any conflicts.)

Step 2: Identify any conflicts that could affect your workouts getting completed. Look at your work schedule this week. Do you have to travel this week? Are there any meetings or events you need to be at that could be overlapping a scheduled workout? Now look at your family calendar. What family stuff is going on this week? Do you have a family event or activity going on this week? Do you have a date with a significant other? Do your kids have activities or events this week? What conflicts present themselves?

Step 3: Drag and move your workouts around any conflicts that you face this week. (It is ok to do resistance training workouts on consecutive days if you have to in order to get them in. Ideally, you want to have a rest day between them when possible. It is also ok to do a resistance training workout and a cardio workout on the same day.)

Step 4: Plan out what time of day you will be doing each workout. (In the morning before work, during lunch, after work, on your day off. . .)

Plan Out Your Meals

What I have found to be the most successful way of keeping myself honest to a healthy eating plan throughout the week is meal prepping at the beginning of the week. You must plan out what you're going to eat throughout the week, and prepare it before the week starts. This helps set you up for success. So for example, if I know that every day for breakfast (or for one of my early morning snacks) I'm going to have two hard-boiled eggs and a banana, then on Sunday I'll purchase it, prepare it, and get it ready for the entire week. Meal prepping like this at the beginning of the week, for as many meals and snacks as you can, will help you succeed.

Step 1: In the first chart below, write out everything you plan to eat for your meals and snacks for the upcoming week. (If you are like me and eat the same thing for breakfast every day and repeat snacks often, this will not take very long.) As you fill this out for the week, be sure to write down any planned dinners out, work-related lunches or other meals, events, happy hours, etc.

Step 2: Look over the meals and snacks you planned out for the week and use the second chart to create your grocery list.

Step 3: Get your groceries for the week.

Step 4: Cook/prepare all of your meals for the week.

Meals / Snacks					
	Breakfast	AM Snack (optional)	Lunch	PM Snack (optional)	Dinner
Monday					
Tuesday					
Wednesday					
Thursday					
Friday					
Saturday					
Sunday					

Grocery List
1.
2.
3.
4.
5.
6.
7.
8.
9.
10.

Week 3
Function Better Through Functional Training

Do you live to exercise? If you're like most people, you probably say no to that question. A good workout can sometimes turn your whole day around, but we're still not racing to get to the gym. If we're really honest, we would probably say that we don't live to exercise, we exercise to improve our quality of life.

What is Functional Training?

The best description of functional training is it is made up of the exercises that helps you do daily activities easier and safer.

Let's say there is a gym fanatic who is just getting home after a great workout. For the sake of this hypothetical story, we will call him John. John had a great workout today! He left the gym feeling stronger than he has all year! He did more weight on bench press than he ever has. He felt really strong on the seated row machine, and he finished by getting a great pump from many sets on the seated curl machine. He gets home from the gym, and his little boy runs over to hug him. John bends over to pick up his three-year-old son, and when he does, he throws his back out. Now he can't stand up straight and will spend the rest of the weekend on the couch.

John is really strong, but all the strength in the world is not going to be of any value to you if you don't know how to use it. John's muscles don't know how to work together. Most of the exercises he does use only one muscle group at a time and just go in one direction.

I've always believed that your training should resemble what you are training for. What do you want to gain from your workouts? Do you want to move better or be able to be more active without pain? Do you want less back pain? Do you want more flexibility? These are good examples of what many people desire as a result of training as well as their motivation for exercising in the first place.

In the Make Fitness A Priority Online Training Program, the exercises use your lower body and your upper body while also incorporating your core. By using multiple muscles and multiple ranges of motion, not only are you going to burn a lot more calories but you're going to teach your muscles how to work together. This will make you stronger and better at performing daily activities.

Action Steps:

Take a second to go back to Week 1 and read what you wrote as your WHY. What do you want to gain from your workouts? Do your workouts resemble what you are training for?

_____

_____

_____

Mindset: Overcoming the "I'm Too Tired" Obstacle

An obstacle that can get in the way of you getting your workout in is simply feeling too tired to work out. Feeling too tired or unmotivated to work out is a common issue and does not mean you are lazy. There are many factors that can contribute to this and also many solutions to overcome it.

When overcoming this obstacle, here are a few things to think about:

How active are you?

If you have a sedentary job and live a sedentary life, then your body will not give you the same amount of energy as an active person. Your body only makes what you need and use. If you start getting more active throughout the day consistently, then you will probably find that you have more energy. So the first step is to get more active.

If you feel like you are an active person and still lack the energy you need, then here are some more things to consider.

How much sleep are you getting?

If you are tired a lot during the day, one reason could be that you are not getting enough sleep. Our bodies need sleep to recover physically and mentally after long days. Do you struggle with getting enough sleep? Try going to bed closer to sundown and waking closer to sunup. Our bodies' natural clock functions better on this schedule, so this little change could have you feeling much more rested.

Are you drinking enough water?

Dehydration can play a role in feeling tired. Water is our bodies' most important nutrient, and many of us don't consume as much as we need to every day. Symptoms of dehydration can include feeling tired, weak, and dizzy. Make sure you are drinking half your body weight in ounces every day.

What kind of fuel are you putting in the tank?

When we feel lethargic during the day, it could be a result of the low quality of food we are eating. If we eat like crap, we are going to feel like crap. That's just the way it goes. If you aren't eating quality food then you will often feel bad effects. Try cutting out all processed foods, fast foods, and cut down on sugar.

Are you setting yourself up to fail?

The last thing I would consider, if you are struggling to find energy to get your workouts in, is if you are scheduling your workouts at a time when you will have energy left to do it. If you have a stressful job, or a job that takes a lot out of you, then you may not have any energy left to work out after work. It may make more sense for you to work out in the early morning before work, or on your days off. If you are someone who plans to work out after work, but constantly find yourself talking yourself out of it, you need to find a new time to work out. If after work is the only option you have, you need to increase your accountability to it somehow. You could get a workout partner, hire a personal trainer, or find a class after work to attend. All of these ideas add a level of accountability that could help you get more consistent. You could also try moving your workouts to days that aren't as busy. If you know that Tuesdays are always your busiest or most stressful days of the week, then it will probably be the hardest to work out after work that day. Maybe Mondays or Fridays are lighter days that wouldn't exhaust you too much for an evening workout.

Action Steps:

Do you struggle with the "I'm too tired" obstacle? How does it affect you?

_____

_____

_____

How can you incorporate these tips to help you overcome it in the future?

_____

_____

_____

Nutrition: Healthy Eating Guidelines Part 2

Last week we covered three healthy habits for you to begin following. How have you done with these new habits? This week we will add just two new habits.

1. Log Your Food

Many people are against keeping track of calories and would prefer to keep track of macros, and that's fine. The fact is that when we are struggling to get results, a lot of times the reason we are stuck is that we are underestimating how many calories we are consuming, and overestimating how many calories we are burning. In order to burn stored body fat, we have to burn more calories than we consume. There is no way around that. By logging your food, you will learn exactly how many calories you are eating, and know if you are eating too much or not enough.

After logging for a few weeks, you will have a good understanding of how much you are eating and won't necessarily have to keep it up. Whenever you hit a plateau in your progress, you can always start logging again to make sure you are still consuming the right amount of food and that your portion sizes haven't grown.

Great food logs: www.myfitnesspal.com, loseit.com, and myplate at livestrong.com

2. Don't Be Misled When Reading Labels

When I first learned how to count calories and read labels, my favorite product was zero-calorie butter spray. I used it on everything. I used a lot of it. I would actually unscrew the cap and just pour it on my food sometimes. Why not? There are no calories in it, right? That means I can have as much of it as I want without any consequences, right? Wrong!

If you look closer at the label you will see that just one spray is a serving, and there are actually well over 1,000 servings in that little bottle. Why in the world would they do that? They do that because one spray is about 0.9 calories, which they can call zero calories. There are actually over 1,000 calories in the bottle. Many zero-calorie or low-calorie food products are like this. Be sure to pay close attention to the label!

Actions Steps:

How will you incorporate these new guidelines this week?

_____

_____

_____

How can you ensure success in adding these new healthy habits?

_____

_____

_____

Training: Find a Way, Not an Excuse

When doing online personal training, there is one excuse that I have found that pops up from time to time, and that is the "I don't have all the right equipment to do this workout" excuse.

Here are just a few scenarios where this can become a problem:

- It's crowded in the gym, and all of the equipment you need for your workout is being used.

- You are doing a home workout and don't have all of the equipment that you need to do a few of the exercises.

- You are traveling and doing your workout in a small hotel fitness center, and there is limited equipment to use.

When these situations pop up, you can't let them be an excuse to skip your workout. You have to develop a "no matter what" mentality. Sometimes you may have to make a little bit of an adjustment, and it won't look exactly the same as it does on your workout online. Maybe you don't have kettlebells available to use in some of the exercises, but you can use dumbbells instead. Maybe you don't have a step to step up on, but you can use a bench or stairs. Maybe you don't have a BOSU, but you can still do that same exercise just on the floor. There's always going to be a way that you can do it, you just have to find a way, not an excuse. No matter what the equipment is you're missing, just use your brain and think, "How can I make this as close to what the workout is as safely as possible?"

Sometimes you will have to make adjustments to get your workout in, but you can always find a way. Every time you have to think outside the box and make do with what you have, that voice that says you can't do it gets weaker. Eventually, getting your workout in will be easy no matter what adjustments you have to make on the fly.

Action Steps:

Have you been faced with the "I don't have the right equipment for this workout" obstacle yet? Did you find a way or find an excuse? What would you do differently next time?

_____

_____

_____

Weekly Fitness Evaluation Form

Now, it is time to give yourself a grade for the week. By doing this weekly self-evaluation and asking yourself the questions on this sheet, you will learn how to keep yourself accountable to your fitness plan. Every week you will learn more from doing this evaluation, and before long your fitness plan will become a top priority in your life.

Here is how this works: Answer the questions below, and then grade yourself for the week. If you give yourself an A+, awesome! All you have to do is just keep it up. If you don't give yourself an A+, ask yourself what went wrong. What obstacles got in your way? How can you overcome these obstacles in the future? These questions will help you when setting yourself up for next week's success.

First, let's start with what you did well . . .

Name three things you are proud of after this week:

1._____

2._____

3._____

Mindset

How was your energy this week? If it was low, did you get enough sleep? Did you drink enough water? What other factors could've affected your energy?

_____

_____

_____

How did you feel during your workouts this week? (Ex: strong or weak, athletic or uncoordinated, tired or energetic)

_____

_____

_____

How was your motivation this week? Was it easy to get your workouts in or challenging? Was it easy to stick to the healthy guidelines or challenging?

_____

_____

_____

What grade do you give your mindset for this week? ___

Nutrition

Did you throw out the temptations and replace them with healthier options?

_____

_____

_____

Did you follow a meal plan? Did you get all your meals in? Did you drink enough water?

_____

_____

_____

Did you have any treats or cheats? If yes, what were your cheat meals? Were they intentional or unplanned?

_____

_____

_____

What grade do you give your nutrition this week? ___

Training

Did you get all of your workouts in this week (resistance training and cardio training)? If your answer is no, which workouts did you miss/skip? Why didn't you get them in?

_____

_____

_____

Did you need to make modifications to any exercises this week? If yes, which exercises, and why/how did you modify them?

_____

_____

_____

What grade do you give your workouts this week? ___

You will use your answers to the questions in this evaluation in the next section, "Set Yourself Up for Success."

Set Yourself Up for Success
in Week 4

Now, it's time to set yourself up for success for the upcoming week. Your fitness goals are no different than anything else you want to accomplish in life. If you don't have a plan, then you might as well plan to fail. The action steps in this form are designed to help you reach your goals in the week ahead.

The first thing we're going to do is overcome the biggest excuse that we always make: "I don't have time." We love this excuse, and it is the easiest one to use.

Make Time

We are going to overcome this excuse right now by making time. The way you make time is scheduling your workouts.

Step 1: Go to your online training program and click on your calendar. I have scheduled your workouts out for the week, but you have the ability to drag and move them to whatever day you'd like. (Not doing one of my online training programs? No problem. You can use your phone calendar or your desk calendar, and just move your workouts around any conflicts.)

Step 2: Identify any conflicts that could affect your workouts getting completed. Look at your work schedule this week. Do you have to travel this week? Are there any meetings or events you need to be at that could be overlapping a scheduled workout? Now look at your family calendar. What family stuff is going on this week? Do you have a family event or activity going on this week? Do you have a date with a significant other? Do your kids have activities or events this week? What conflicts present themselves?

Step 3: Drag and move your workouts around any conflicts that you face this week. (It is ok to do resistance training workouts on consecutive days if you have to in order to get them in. Ideally, you want to have a rest day between them when possible. It is also ok to do a resistance training workout and a cardio workout on the same day.)

Step 4: Plan out what time of day you will be doing each workout. (In the morning before work, during lunch, after work, on your day off...)

Plan Out Your Meals

What I have found to be the most successful way of keeping myself honest to a healthy eating plan throughout the week is meal prepping at the beginning of the week. You must plan out what you're going to eat throughout the week, and prepare it before the week starts. This helps set you up for success. So for example, if I know that every day for breakfast (or for one of my early morning snacks) I'm going to have two hard-boiled eggs and a banana, then on Sunday I'll purchase it, prepare it, and get it ready for the entire week. Meal prepping like this at the beginning of the week, for as many meals and snacks as you can, will help you succeed.

Step 1: In the first chart below, write out everything you plan to eat for your meals and snacks for the upcoming week. (If you are like me and eat the same thing for breakfast every day and repeat snacks often, this will not take very long.) As you fill this out for the week, be sure to write down any planned dinners out, work-related lunches or other meals, events, happy hours, etc.

Step 2: Look over the meals and snacks you planned out for the week and use the second chart to create your grocery list.

Step 3: Get your groceries for the week.

Step 4: Cook/prepare all of your meals for the week.

Meals / Snacks					
	Breakfast	AM Snack (optional)	Lunch	PM Snack (optional)	Dinner
Monday					
Tuesday					
Wednesday					
Thursday					
Friday					
Saturday					
Sunday					

Grocery List
1.
2.
3.
4.
5.
6.
7.
8.
9.
10.

Week 4
Failing Is Not the End . . .
Failing Is Inevitable

When you think of the words *fail* and *goals*, a phrase that may come to mind is, New Year's resolutions. Sharing your New Year's resolutions is not as powerful as it once was because everyone expects you to fail. This is not an anti-goal-setting rant. Everybody should have goals and set goals regularly. The purpose of this is to take a stand against the negativity that comes with those three words: New Year's resolutions. Have you ever heard a positive story about a person who successfully kept their New Year's resolution? Probably not. I bet you've heard at least a dozen stories about New Year's resolution fails though.

There is so much negativity around New Year's resolutions that most people refuse to make them at all. They feel it's just a waste of time, that they are doomed to fail anyway, so why even bother. They feel resolutions are just promises we make to ourselves every year and don't follow through on. How sad is that? We don't even believe the words coming out of our own mouths anymore.

Who determines our failure on the goals we set? If we miss one workout, or eat one thing that isn't part of our plan, does that mean we're failures? Are your standards for yourself really to be perfect? If that is the case, then I hate to have to tell you this, but your goals are unrealistic.

I admire and appreciate the belief you have in yourself to set the bar that high. I attack most things in my life with a "losing is not an option" mentality as well, but you have to give yourself a break. You are human, and you are going to fail from time to time. But the story doesn't have to end there.

Reaching your fitness goals (especially your long-term ones) does not come without making mistakes. No one can be expected to be perfect. You are human and mistakes are allowed.

I have good news though. Failing is actually good. It is what makes us stronger and leads us to long-term success.

Success doesn't come by never failing. Success comes from learning how to get back on track each time you make a mistake. Failure does not define you, nor does it stop you from reaching your goals. What defines you is how you respond after you fail.

Action Steps: Getting Back Up

What mistakes have you made in the first three weeks of your fitness program?

_____

_____

_____

How did you respond after failing?

_____

_____

_____

Your fitness journey doesn't have to end just because you failed. Failing is inevitable. Failing does not define you. What defines you is how you respond to failing. The next time you make a mistake, remind yourself that it's what you do next that counts.

Mindset: Overcoming the "I'm Too Busy" Excuse

In all of my years in fitness, I believe that this is the biggest obstacle that most of us face in making fitness a priority in our lives. We have other priorities in our lives also, like our family and our jobs, and when they demand a lot of our time, fitness is usually what loses balance. If you are struggling to overcome this roadblock, here are a few tips that have helped my clients and myself over the years.

To make your workouts a priority you have to put them in your calendar.

You have important things happening all the time with your job and your family that you never miss because they are always in your schedule. You have to start treating your workouts the same way. Schedule out every workout (day and time) and mark them on your calendar. Schedule your workouts as far out as possible. Once your workouts are in your calendar, you can no longer use the "I don't have time" excuse because you just made time.

Check your schedule for conflicts regularly.

At the beginning of every week, look at your schedule to make sure there are no conflicts popping up that will get in the way of your scheduled workouts. Look at both your work calendar and your family calendar. Are there any work conflicts (late meetings, events, happy hours, travel, etc.) that could get in the way? Are there any family conflicts (kids' activities, birthdays, anniversaries, date nights, etc.) that could get in the way? When conflicts come up that stop you from being able to do a workout, don't just cancel your workout, reschedule it to a better time. Reschedule all workouts that have conflicts before the week starts.

Does the workout routine you're doing make sense for your current lifestyle?

Sometimes when someone says that they are "too busy" to work out, it really means they are too busy to work out like they used to. Our lives are constantly changing. We get promotions, we have busy seasons, and family events like kids' activities come and go. Just because we don't have as much time to dedicate to fitness at a certain time of year doesn't mean we can't still make fitness a priority. Maybe you don't have the time to spend an hour and a half at the gym every day like you once did, but you can still reap great benefits from training for 45 minutes two or three days per week. Make sure what you are doing makes sense for the life you are currently living.

Action Steps:

Have you been scheduling your workouts? How well have you been able to reschedule your workouts around conflicts? What can you do better?

_____

_____

_____

Nutrition: Healthy Eating Guidelines
Part 3

Last week we covered two healthy habits for you to begin following. How have you done with these new habits? This week we will add two new habits.

1. Avoid Products With Too Many Ingredients

When someone starts logging food for the first time, they are usually shocked when they learn how many calories they've been eating. Another thing that they usually discover is that they are consuming way too much fat and not nearly enough protein. In our defense, we are victims of the convenient fast food day and age we live in. A common side effect of this high fat discovery is low-fat and fat-free shopping. There are many low-fat or fat-free snack options available these days, but are they healthy? That depends. Let's take a look at the ingredient list of a fat-free devil's food cookie snack option.

The first ingredient is . . . sugar (not off to a good start, let's see where this goes from here), unbleached enriched flour [wheat flour, niacin, reduced iron, thiamine mononitrate (vitamin B1)], riboflavin (vitamin B2), folic acid, corn syrup, high fructose corn syrup, cocoa (processed with alkali), skim milk, gelatin, glycerin, leavening (baking soda and/or sodium acid pyrophosphate and/or calcium phosphate).

Let's pause right there for a second. Don't you just love it when it says "and/or" in the ingredient list? How are they not sure what they put in their product? Does this bother anyone else?

Ok, back to the ingredient list: emulsifiers (mono and diglycerides, soy lecithin), cornstarch, chocolate, modified cornstarch, salt, potassium sorbate added to preserve freshness, artificial flavor.

I'm not going to lie to you, I don't know what many of these words are or even how to pronounce them correctly. I feel like they are much better suited to be in a spelling bee than on the back of a product I'm about to consume. This product is just 50 calories, but our bodies do not like processed foods like this.

Plus, we learned from the butter spray last week to always look at the serving size, and the serving size of this product is just one cookie. I can't remember a time that I have only had one cookie, so I know how this would go. Here is a tip for you: If it takes longer to read the ingredient list than it does to eat the product, don't eat it!

If It Sounds Too Good to Be True . . . It Probably Is

Who knew nutritious could be so delicious? This is something I remember reading before on a box of reduced sugar chocolate chip cookies. These chocolate chip cookies looked good on the box, and on the box it said that they taste just as good as original cookies. Guaranteed or your money back it even said.

Remember that if it sounds too good to be true, it is.

If you look at the ingredient list, you'll probably see many red flags, the first being that the ingredient list is a mile long. The second would be that the list contains words like sucrose, dextrose, fructose, polyglycerides and monoglycerides, polydextrose, and of course, high fructose corn syrup. All these words are different ways of describing sugar.

There are many different types of sugar, and when you put all the different types of sugar on there, it allows you to not make "sugar" the number one ingredient on the list. This is almost as scandalous as the zero-calorie butter spray, huh? Always remember, if it sounds too good to be true, it probably is!

Action Step:

Begin using these tips as you do your grocery shopping this week.

What foods have you purchased in the past that these tips can keep you away from?

_____

_____

_____

Training: Good Days & Bad Days

When you start working out on a regular basis and working out becomes a permanent part of your life and not just a temporary thing, you notice that there are good days and bad days. Some days you will feel great about your workout—you will feel like you have endless amounts of energy and feel very strong. Other days you just won't feel like you have it. You might feel tired or weak or just not into it.

Some days how you feel will make total sense to you. You may feel like a superhero during Monday's workout, and when you think about it, you realize you ate great over the weekend, got caught up on sleep, and have just been in a great mood. Then on Friday, you really struggle to do your workout, and you realize it has been a very stressful week at work and you are just exhausted. These kinds of days are easy to go through because they make sense.

There will be days that you feel good or bad, and it just doesn't add up to you. You feel like you have been really dialed in on everything from what you eat to getting enough sleep, but when it's time for your workout, you just struggle. Then on the flip side, you will have days when you are undisciplined on your food and sleep, but then feel stronger than ever in your workout.

Sometimes it's hard to figure out what causes these days, and trying to solve that mystery will make your head hurt. The trick is just to keep going forward. Embrace the good days. Be thankful for them and give them all you have. When the unexpected bad days pop up think of them as opportunities to grow. Finishing strong on these challenging days will make the good days come around more often.

These ups and downs are normal, and everyone goes through it. Never let a bad day break your spirit.

Action Step:

Have you had an unexpected good day or bad day on one of your workouts yet? How did you handle it? What can you do differently next time?

_____

_____

_____

Weekly Fitness Evaluation Form

Now, it is time to give yourself a grade for the week. By doing this weekly self-evaluation and asking yourself the questions on this sheet, you will learn how to keep yourself accountable to your fitness plan. Every week you will learn more from doing this evaluation, and before long your fitness plan will become a top priority in your life.

Here is how this works: Answer the questions below, and then grade yourself for the week. If you give yourself an A+, awesome! All you have to do is just keep it up. If you don't give yourself an A+, ask yourself what went wrong. What obstacles got in your way? How can you overcome these obstacles in the future? These questions will help you when setting yourself up for next week's success.

First, let's start with what you did well . . .

Name three things you are proud of after this week:

1._____

2._____

3._____

Mindset

How was your energy this week? If it was low, did you get enough sleep? Did you drink enough water? What other factors could've affected your energy?

_____

_____

_____

How did you feel during your workouts this week? (Ex: strong or weak, athletic or uncoordinated, tired or energetic)

_____

_____

_____

How was your motivation this week? Was it easy to get your workouts in or challenging? Was it easy to stick to the healthy guidelines or challenging?

_____

_____

_____

What grade do you give your mindset for this week? ___

Nutrition

Did you throw out the temptations and replace them with healthier options?

_____

_____

_____

Did you follow a meal plan? Did you get all your meals in? Did you drink enough water?

_____

_____

_____

Did you have any treats or cheats? If yes, what were your cheat meals? Were they intentional or unplanned?

_____

_____

_____

What grade do you give your nutrition this week? ___

Training

Did you get all of your workouts in this week (resistance training and cardio training)? If your answer is no, which workouts did you miss/skip? Why didn't you get them in?

_____

_____

_____

Did you need to make modifications to any exercises this week? If yes, which exercises, and why/how did you modify them?

_____

_____

_____

What grade do you give your workouts this week? ___

You will use your answers to the questions in this evaluation in the next section, "Set Yourself Up for Success."

Set Yourself Up for Success
in Week 5

Now, it's time to set yourself up for success for the upcoming week. Your fitness goals are no different than anything else you want to accomplish in life. If you don't have a plan, then you might as well plan to fail. The action steps in this form are designed to help you reach your goals in the week ahead.

The first thing we're going to do is overcome the biggest excuse that we always make: "I don't have time." We love this excuse, and it is the easiest one to use.

Make Time

We are going to overcome this excuse right now by making time. The way you make time is scheduling your workouts.

Step 1: Go to your online training program and click on your calendar. I have scheduled your workouts out for the week, but you have the ability to drag and move them to whatever day you'd like. (Not doing one of my online training programs? No problem. You can use your phone calendar or your desk calendar, and just move your workouts around any conflicts.)

Step 2: Identify any conflicts that could affect your workouts getting completed. Look at your work schedule this week. Do you have to travel this week? Are there any meetings or events you need to be at that could be overlapping a scheduled workout? Now look at your family calendar. What family stuff is going on this week? Do you have a family event or activity going on this week? Do you have a date with a significant other? Do your kids have activities or events this week? What conflicts present themselves?

Step 3: Drag and move your workouts around any conflicts that you face this week. (It is ok to do resistance training workouts on consecutive days if you have to in order to get them in. Ideally, you want to have a rest day between them when possible. It is also ok to do a resistance training workout and a cardio workout on the same day.)

Step 4: Plan out what time of day you will be doing each workout. (In the morning before work, during lunch, after work, on your day off. . .)

Plan Out Your Meals

What I have found to be the most successful way of keeping myself honest to a healthy eating plan throughout the week is meal prepping at the beginning of the week. You must plan out what you're going to eat throughout the week, and prepare it before the week starts. This helps set you up for success. So for example, if I know that every day for breakfast (or for one of my early morning snacks) I'm going to have two hard-boiled eggs and a banana, then on Sunday I'll purchase it, prepare it, and get it ready for the entire week. Meal prepping like this at the beginning of the week, for as many meals and snacks as you can, will help you succeed.

Step 1: In the first chart below, write out everything you plan to eat for your meals and snacks for the upcoming week. (If you are like me and eat the same thing for breakfast every day and repeat snacks often, this will not take very long.) As you fill this out for the week, be sure to write down any planned dinners out, work-related lunches or other meals, events, happy hours, etc.

Step 2: Look over the meals and snacks you planned out for the week and use the second chart to create your grocery list.

Step 3: Get your groceries for the week.

Step 4: Cook/prepare all of your meals for the week.

Meals / Snacks					
	Breakfast	AM Snack (optional)	Lunch	PM Snack (optional)	Dinner
Monday					
Tuesday					
Wednesday					
Thursday					
Friday					
Saturday					
Sunday					

Grocery List
1.
2.
3.
4.
5.
6.
7.
8.
9.
10.

Week 5
A Letter to My Obstacles

There is no doubt that you are the favorite in this competition, and I am the underdog. You are a proven champion, and most people will bet on you. You can be very intimidating if I allow you to be. Just like Muhammad Ali, you have the ability to beat many of your opponents before the match even starts. I know I can't ignore you. I know you will not just go away. You are what stands between me and my goals. The sooner I get past you, the sooner I will be back on the path toward success.

Many people before me have failed to get past you. Why is that? Did they stop believing in themselves? Was the fear of failure too much for them to take? Did they allow other people's opinions to shake their confidence?

All of these victories have made you a little too cocky. It's my turn now, and I don't think you realize who you are dealing with! Sure, you may win a few rounds. You may even knock me down a few times. I will probably fail over and over again. But I won't quit! I am stubborn! I have the resiliency to keep getting back up. You will not break my spirit no matter how much pain you put me through!

My body will get exhausted. Every muscle will hurt, and I will begin to hear voices pleading with me to throw in the towel. Quitting will start to seem like an easy option. I could come up with many excuses why I can't do it. I could find several people to point my finger at and blame for my failure. It would be easy to validate coming up short. I have bad news for you, though . . . I never do anything the easy way!

I know I will not pass you if I quit. If I quit, I fail. Therefore, quitting is not an option! I will find a way to keep going. It may start to seem like I am moving in slow motion . . . but I will keep going! Eventually I will flip the switch in my head, and instead of focusing on how much farther I still have to go, I will start focusing on how far I've already come! I will realize that I've come way too far to stop now!

This is very important to me, and I've put in a lot of hard work to get here. Not everyone believed I could do it. I've been laughed at, and I've been criticized. There have always been people who didn't believe in me, and there always will be. I didn't get to where I am by listening to the naysayers. Just because others quit, doesn't mean I have to! Just because others decided they couldn't do it, doesn't mean I can't!

I have prepared well for this moment, and my preparation has made me strong. I have learned from my mistakes. I have strengthened my weaknesses. I have surrounded myself with the right type of people. I understand that no one can do this for me. It is all up to me now. I will not quit! I will not let up UNTIL I WIN!!!

Action Steps:

When we face an obstacle we have two choices: either we can overcome the obstacle or the obstacle can overcome us. What is your biggest obstacle right now?

_____

_____

_____

Mindset: How to Be a Donut Slayer

In my book, *Make Fitness a Priority: How to Win the Fight Against Excuses*, I talk a lot about the obstacles we face in fitness and how we use these obstacles as excuses. Excuses like "I'm too busy," "I'm too tired," "I have to travel for work," "I have to be at my kids' activities," etc. We can see these obstacles coming from a mile away, and we can come up with a plan of attack well in advance to overcome them. With just a little discipline, overcoming these obstacles becomes a piece of cake over time.

The toughest obstacles to overcome are the ones that are unexpected and you can't plan for. Life throws us a curveball from time to time that forces us to throw the game plan out the window. In the fitness world, I like to refer to these curveballs as donuts. I call them donuts because donuts have the power to be either the best or the worst things ever created. They can be a great cheat meal reward at the end of a tough week of workouts, or they can cause your meal plan to spiral out of control.

Some of my best workouts have come when I have had to change my plans at the last minute and adapt to the situation. Having to change your plans at the last minute doesn't have to be such a bad thing. When life throws you one of these curveballs, as it for sure will from time to time, it is up to you how you respond. I am going to teach you how to become a donut slayer.

The key to becoming a donut slayer is simple: You have to develop a "No Matter What" mindset! "I'm going to get my workout in *no matter what*. I'm going to stick to my meal plan *no matter what*." Where there is desire, there is always a way.

The next time the unexpected occurs, the first thing you need to do is remind yourself that you have at your disposal a very powerful tool for solving any dilemma. That powerful tool is your own brain. To come up with a solution to any donut, all you have to do is use it. Your mind is always more powerful than your problems.

Here are some examples of some of the top DONUTS I see my clients face on a regular basis.

Bad Weather Donut:

Situation: You wake up early, planning to go for a morning run, and open the door to discover it is raining outside.

Solution: If you're changing your plans for an outdoor workout just because it's raining, then I would recommend asking yourself why. Is there a law against working out in the rain? I wouldn't suggest running in a lightning storm or a blizzard, but if it's just rain, then what's stopping you? You don't really believe that you will melt, do you?

I personally find a rainy workout to be very empowering! Think about it. By not letting the weather stop you, you are overcoming an obstacle that most people chose to avoid. Don't you think that is something that will make you stronger, and make getting future workouts in even easier. If you have never experienced a run in the rain, I would highly recommend it.

I'm so used to it now that rain doesn't even phase me. When I get up to go for an early morning run and it's raining, the only thing that changes is that I wear a hat to keep the rain out of my eyes. Think about it like this: the worst thing that will happen is that you will get wet. Weren't you planning to take a shower after your workout anyway?

Sick Kid Donut:

Situation: You get a call from your kid's teacher and find out that your child has been spending the morning throwing up all over the other kids.

Solution: Hopefully when this happens you are able to work from home for your job and don't have to take the day off. As far as your workout goes, this isn't really a big deal. All this means is that you will have to cancel your plans to go to the gym and simply do your workout at home near your child. If your child is really sick, you will probably have the most success splitting your workout into small chunks of just five to fifteen minutes.

Extra Work Donut:

Situation: Your boss is nice enough to let you know after lunch that the deadline for your current project is now tomorrow morning. Finishing that project and getting your boss off your back is now going to be your top priority.

Solution: Hopefully when this happens you are told about it at least the day before, but sometimes things come up that day that make you have to stay at work longer. The way I normally handle this dilemma is to reschedule this workout as an extra workout later in the week, probably as an early morning workout or lunchtime workout. Having a two-workout day can catch you up, so you still get all your workouts in.

Of course, if it is already the end of the week, this won't be an option. If this is something that happens on a regular basis with your job, the best plan of attack is to start scheduling your workouts in the morning before you go to work. That way, no matter what fires get started at work during the day, you will still get your workout in.

Leaving Town Donut:

Situation: Your boss tells you on Monday morning that he needs you to travel to Seattle to put out a few fires for your company.

Solution: Usually when you are traveling for work, you know about it in advance, so you can adjust your workout schedule to accommodate it. If this is a surprise work trip that comes with short notice, you will have to find a way to get your workouts in while you're gone. Just because the location is changing doesn't mean your goal has to. You can get a good workout in anywhere.

If you are a member at a big national gym, then there might be one nearby. If you're staying in a hotel, there will probably be a fitness center that you can use. If there isn't a fitness center, there will probably be some stairs, and you don't need any equipment to do bodyweight exercises. You may still be busy with work meetings and such, but there are plenty of options for you to still get quick workouts in while you're there.

I Forgot Donut:

Situation 1: You get to the locker room to change and realize you forgot workout clothes or gym shoes.

Solution 1: What a dilemma this can be. I have been known to have my clients workout in jeans, dress shoes, sandals, or even barefoot in the past. I would do this because I want to help instill the "No Matter What" mindset in my clients. But sometimes this is a mistake that can't be worked around, and you will have no choice but to either workout out at home or take an unscheduled trip home.

A good tip to help avoid this mistake from messing up future workouts is to put an emergency gym bag in your car. Put a spare set of gym clothes, shoes, gloves, music, and whatever else you might need in the bag. That way, the next time you forget something you are covered.

Situation 2: You are all ready for your workout, take one step out of the locker room, and realize your iPod is dead!

Solution 2: For me, this is a nightmare. Sometimes you need some help from guys like Metallica or AC/DC to get into workout mode. When you're used to having your own music during your workout, it can seem like a huge obstacle when you have to go without it. Usually, once you get started, you won't even realize that you don't have it, but sometimes it can make your workout seem really boring (especially if you're doing cardio).

One tip that might help you power through is to shorten some things up. For your cardio workouts, do interval training instead of an endurance workout. You can get the same results and finish faster. You could also split your workout into multiple machines for shorter periods of time instead of just one machine for a long period of time. By raising the intensity, you can get the same results with a shorter workout.

Un-Motivated Donut:

Situation: You have been killing your workouts lately, but it has been a very long and stressful week. You get to the gym and just don't feel like working out at all today.

Solution: We all have days like this! Some days you just don't feel like working out. What drives us to put in the work is our WHY fuel. Start by reminding yourself what your goals are and why you are putting in this work.

On days like this, I like to follow the ten-minute rule. Tell yourself that you have to do at least ten minutes. Usually by the time you are ten minutes into your workout, you will have been able to wrap your mind around it, and it won't be hard to keep going. If after ten minutes you end up stopping, then you at least did ten minutes, which is better than nothing.

Eating Out Donut:

Situation: Your company's president is in town for a surprise visit and you have to go to dinner with him and your boss.

Solution: Many people are scared to eat out when trying to follow a meal plan, but there is really no reason to be scared. You first need to decide if you are going to follow your plan or deviate from it. If you are going to make this a cheat meal, then just enjoy it! Don't feel guilty or beat yourself up about it while you are there. Just get back on track on the very next meal, don't let this one meal turn into multiple.

If you are going to stick to your plan, the first rule is to not go to the restaurant starving. Some people like to starve themselves all day to save calories for this meal, but that is a bad idea. All that will do is set you up to binge on bread, chips, or other things. Get all of your meals in throughout the day as you normally would.

When you look at the menu, start by choosing your protein first, and then pick the rest of the meal based on your protein choice. If you order a steak that is protein and fat, you will want leaner sides like vegetables. If you choose a leaner protein like chicken or fish, you can have a starchy carb like a potato or rice. When you order, keep in mind that you are the boss. Don't be afraid to ask for substitutions. The last thing to keep in mind is alcohol. If you want to have wine or a few beers with your meal, you want a lean meal with fewer starches.

These are just a few examples of donuts. There are obviously many more where these came from. The next time one of these unexpected obstacles pop up, remind yourself that your mind is more powerful than your problems, and you have the tools you need to come up with a solution to any donut.

Action Step: Your Donuts

What donuts have you faced since starting your workout program?

_____

_____

_____

What solutions can help you overcome these donuts in the future?

_____

_____

_____

Nutrition: Healthy Eating Guidelines
Part 4

Last week we covered two healthy habits for you to begin following. How have you done with these new habits? This week we will add two new habits.

1. Count Quality, Not Just Quantity (Eat Real Food)

When we start logging food, we tend to discover a lot of what I call convenience choices. I'm referring to the 100-calorie snack pack options that always catch our attention when we shop. People come to me confused all the time saying, "You said all I had to do was burn more calories than I took in and I'd lose weight! I'm positive I'm taking in less calories than I'm burning, so why am I not losing weight?"

When you look at the big picture of calories in versus calories out, you have every right to be a little confused. If you are taking in less than you are burning, then you should be burning stored body fat, right? Unfortunately, every person's body responds differently, and it's not always that simple. What you have to factor in is that not every calorie is the same. At least not according to our bodies.

Think about this: If I were to build a 500-pound house out of bricks and another 500-pound house out of tissues, would they both withstand the same amount of wind? Of course not. Obviously, the integrity of both houses would be different. Our bodies react the same way toward the food we eat. Processed foods with too many ingredients can really hurt our results. It is true that in order to burn stored body fat we have to burn more calories than we consume; however, it is just as important that we count quality and not just quantity.

Whenever we modify a food over and over again until it is just a shred of its former self, it is no longer a healthy choice. So what should you eat? Fruits, vegetables, lean meats, eggs, oats, nuts, etc. These foods have not been altered and have not been broken down. If you look at the back of a bag of almonds, under ingredients it will just say almonds. If you look at the ingredients of oatmeal, it will say rolled oats. You get the idea. It's time to cut down on processed foods and start eating real food.

2. Don't Abuse Your Cheat Meals

I am a firm believer in cheat meals. I do my best when I allow myself to cheat on my meal plan from time to time. It helps me control my cravings, and it keeps me from going insane. However, cheat meals can hurt your results if you abuse them.

When you first start eating a healthier diet, you are probably cutting out a good amount of sugar and fat that was in your everyday diet before. Let's not lie, it's not easy to say goodbye to these things. The longer you stick to your meal plan, the easier it is, but it is a sacrifice at first. For me, saying that I would never have a cheat meal again is unrealistic and a recipe for future failure.

Having a weekly or bi-weekly cheat meal can help you stick to your healthy meal plan much easier. It is also just as important to stay disciplined to the cheat meal and make sure it is just one meal or snack (a cheat or treat). Sometimes a cheat meal can become a cheat day, and then a cheat weekend. When this happens, you erase all of the hard work you did during the week. To have the best chance of success is to be intentional with everything you eat, even when you eat a cheat meal. Plan out your treat or cheat ahead of time, and then stick to your plan.

Action Steps:

How can you incorporate these new guidelines in your life as new habits?

_____

_____

_____

How could these guidelines have helped you in the past?

_____

_____

_____

Training: What's Next?

Wow!! You are almost through five weeks of your six-week workbook already. Have you been doing the Make Fitness A Priority Online Training Program? How have you liked it? How have your workouts been going? What has changed in your life? What new habits and routines have you started, and what bad habits have you stopped? Have you been able to establish a consistent workout schedule? How did you improve from Week 1 to Week 5? I'm sure by now you have learned that making fitness a priority in your life takes work, but with practice you can be just as consistent with it as everything else in your life.

Now that we are down to your last few workouts, it is time to look toward the future. What do you plan to do next? I hope that this program has helped you get into a regular routine, and that there is no doubt in your mind that fitness is going to be a part of your life going forward. If you would like to keep working with me as your online trainer, I would be happy to keep training you. I have several training options that you can choose from here: https://overlandparkfitness.com/online-training/

My recommendation:

Try my **Be Fit...For Life Online Program**. It has two total-body resistance training workouts every week (one home workout and one gym workout), and one creative cardio workout that you do twice. Creative cardio workouts are just as the title describes . . . creative. If you are bored with your cardio workouts, you will love the creative cardio workouts.

It is $24.99 per month, and you can get half off your first month with **promo code: save50**

Action Steps:

Remember this is not just a six-week program . . . this is the first six weeks of fitness being a priority in your life. What do you plan to do for your next workout program? Keep this going! Make sure you have a plan going forward before you're done with your current program.

_____

_____

_____

Exercise

Never

Dies

Weekly Fitness Evaluation Form

Now, it is time to give yourself a grade for the week. By doing this weekly self-evaluation and asking yourself the questions on this sheet, you will learn how to keep yourself accountable to your fitness plan. Every week you will learn more from doing this evaluation, and before long your fitness plan will become a top priority in your life.

Here is how this works: Answer the questions below, and then grade yourself for the week. If you give yourself an A+, awesome! All you have to do is just keep it up. If you don't give yourself an A+, ask yourself what went wrong. What obstacles got in your way? How can you overcome these obstacles in the future? These questions will help you when setting yourself up for next week's success.

First, let's start with what you did well . . .

Name three things you are proud of after this week:

1._____

2._____

3._____

Mindset

How was your energy this week? If it was low, did you get enough sleep? Did you drink enough water? What other factors could've affected your energy?

_____

_____

_____

How did you feel during your workouts this week? (Ex: strong or weak, athletic or uncoordinated, tired or energetic)

_____

_____

_____

How was your motivation this week? Was it easy to get your workouts in or challenging? Was it easy to stick to the healthy guidelines or challenging?

_____

_____

_____

What grade do you give your mindset for this week? ___

Nutrition

Did you throw out the temptations and replace them with healthier options?

_____

_____

_____

Did you follow a meal plan? Did you get all your meals in? Did you drink enough water?

_____

_____

_____

Did you have any treats or cheats? If yes, what were your cheat meals? Were they intentional or unplanned?

_____

_____

_____

What grade do you give your nutrition this week? ___

Training

Did you get all of your workouts in this week (resistance training and cardio training)? If your answer is no, which workouts did you miss/skip? Why didn't you get them in?

_____

_____

_____

Did you need to make modifications to any exercises this week? If yes, which exercises, and why/how did you modify them?

_____

_____

_____

What grade do you give your workouts this week? ___

You will use your answers to the questions in this evaluation in the next section, "Set Yourself Up for Success."

Set Yourself Up for Success
in Week 6

Now, it's time to set yourself up for success for the upcoming week. Your fitness goals are no different than anything else you want to accomplish in life. If you don't have a plan, then you might as well plan to fail. The action steps in this form are designed to help you reach your goals in the week ahead.

The first thing we're going to do is overcome the biggest excuse that we always make: "I don't have time." We love this excuse, and it is the easiest one to use.

Make Time

We are going to overcome this excuse right now by making time. The way you make time is scheduling your workouts.

Step 1: Go to your online training program and click on your calendar. I have scheduled your workouts out for the week, but you have the ability to drag and move them to whatever day you'd like. (Not doing one of my online training programs? No problem. You can use your phone calendar or your desk calendar, and just move your workouts around any conflicts.)

Step 2: Identify any conflicts that could affect your workouts getting completed. Look at your work schedule this week. Do you have to travel this week? Are there any meetings or events you need to be at that could be overlapping a scheduled workout? Now look at your family calendar. What family stuff is going on this week? Do you have a family event or activity going on this week? Do you have a date with a significant other? Do your kids have activities or events this week? What conflicts present themselves?

Step 3: Drag and move your workouts around any conflicts that you face this week. (It is ok to do resistance training workouts on consecutive days if you have to in order to get them in. Ideally, you want to have a rest day between them when possible. It is also ok to do a resistance training workout and a cardio workout on the same day.)

Step 4: Plan out what time of day you will be doing each workout. (In the morning before work, during lunch, after work, on your day off. . .)

Plan Out Your Meals

What I have found to be the most successful way of keeping myself honest to a healthy eating plan throughout the week is meal prepping at the beginning of the week. You must plan out what you're going to eat throughout the week, and prepare it before the week starts. This helps set you up for success. So for example, if I know that every day for breakfast (or for one of my early morning snacks) I'm going to have two hard-boiled eggs and a banana, then on Sunday I'll purchase it, prepare it, and get it ready for the entire week. Meal prepping like this at the beginning of the week, for as many meals and snacks as you can, will help you succeed.

Step 1: In the first chart below, write out everything you plan to eat for your meals and snacks for the upcoming week. (If you are like me and eat the same thing for breakfast every day and repeat snacks often, this will not take very long.) As you fill this out for the week, be sure to write down any planned dinners out, work-related lunches or other meals, events, happy hours, etc.

Step 2: Look over the meals and snacks you planned out for the week and use the second chart to create your grocery list.

Step 3: Get your groceries for the week.

Step 4: Cook/prepare all of your meals for the week.

Meals / Snacks					
	Breakfast	AM Snack (optional)	Lunch	PM Snack (optional)	Dinner
Monday					
Tuesday					
Wednesday					
Thursday					
Friday					
Saturday					
Sunday					

Grocery List
1.
2.
3.
4.
5.
6.
7.
8.
9.
10.

Week 6
Get Off Your BUTs!!

Everyone is capable of accomplishing great things, but we all still have our own obstacles that we face on a regular basis. Recently I realized that there is one obstacle that all of us face. It doesn't matter where we live, how old we are, what nationality we are, what sexual orientation we are, how fit we are, how much money we have, or even what our religion is. We all have the same limiting force that can take away all of our abilities if we let it. It's the size of our but! Some peoples buts are so big that they completely weigh them down! (I'm talking about your "but" not your "butt.")

I would exercise more, but I don't have enough time.

I would eat better, but I don't know how.

I would grow a much more successful business, but it's just too hard.

Sean Stephenson, a motivational speaker and American therapist, wrote a book titled *Get Off Your BUTS*. It's a great book about getting out of your own way. In his book, he says there are three types of BUTS.

First, you have your **BUT Fears**. This but always starts with *but what if* . . . But what if I fail? But what if I look bad?

Second, you have your **BUT Excuses**. This but always starts with *but I don't have the* . . . time, money, resources—whatever it is that you think you're lacking, and if you had it, everything would be fine.

The third but is the worst but of all! It's your **BUT Insecurities**. This but always starts with *but I'm not* . . . But I'm not tall enough. But I'm not fit enough. But I'm not strong enough.

I know I have let these obstacles get the best of me a lot in my past, but over time I have learned that every time you overcome one of these buts, it makes you stronger going forward. I've always believed that the bigger the challenge, the bigger the reward, and when you overcome a big obstacle, it builds your confidence so much that you can overcome any other obstacle that gets in your way.

We let our buts hold us back all of the time! We convince ourselves that are but is so big that it is impossible to overcome. In reality it is just another obstacle, and all we have to do to overcome it is stand up!

Action Steps:

What "buts" did you struggle with during the last five weeks?

_____

_____

_____

How can you overcome them in the future?

_____

_____

_____

Take a stand, and get off your buts!

Mindset: How Strong Is Your Pit Crew?

I don't know if you've heard the news or not, but I am now a three-time World's Toughest Mudder Finisher! In November of 2018, I once again completed this 24-hour obstacle race with my girlfriend, Jess Chadd, by my side as my pit crew. This course is set up as a five-mile loop with 26 obstacles on the course. Competitors of this race are to repeat the five-mile loop as many times as they can in 24 hours. There were 1,570 competitors who started this race, and only 735 total finishers (46% finish rate). I finished in 394th place with a total of 40 miles. This grueling 24-hour challenge taught me a huge life lesson.

Read my short race recap to find out what I learned . . .

It's around 2:00 a.m. on November 11th at World's Toughest Mudder. I've already completed the course several times at this point, and I've just decided to take the penalty lap at the stacks. The stacks, a new obstacle this year, basically consists of climbing up a cargo net that's draped over the top of four shipping containers that are stacked one on top of the other 40-feet high. You climb up the top of the cargo net, walk across the top of the shipping containers, then take a 40-foot jump into some deep water. Most competitors are going to take the same path that I did: bypass the obstacle and go straight to the penalty loop. Partly because when you first walk up to this thing and gaze up to the top, your first response is, "Screw that!" But the biggest reason for the bypass is strategy. It takes a lot of energy to climb up that 40-foot cargo net and the penalty loop is just a short little jog.

Another part of the strategy comes with the cold. It's below freezing outside. It's been below freezing for a couple hours now, so it's really cold. Taking a jump into some cold water that you don't have to take doesn't really make a lot of sense.

So I'm going through the penalty lap, and something starts to happen to me that's never happened to me before in one of these races. As I'm walking, I start to feel like I'm falling asleep, which doesn't make any sense. I know this is a 24-hour race, but I can't be sleepy. I just ran up a ramp in the last obstacle. I'm struggling to keep my eyes open. I try to jump around, wake myself up. I'm still about three miles away from tent city, and after looking around, I also realize that I'm all by myself. Just yesterday morning I was surrounded by 1,500 other competitors at the start line, but now the course is like a ghost town.

I'm freezing. My fingers and toes are going numb. All I can see is the light from my own headlamp and the fog from my breath. I'm cold and alone with only my own thoughts to keep me company. Normally, that would be a really good thing. I'm a pretty positive, upbeat guy. Unfortunately, right now the only thoughts in my head I can hear are, "What the hell am I doing here? Why in the world did I think this was going to be fun? How much more of this can I take? Do I want to take any more of this?"

I keep going, one foot in front of the other, and I make it back to Jess who's waiting for me in tent city. I'm sure she can tell just by my body language that I'm feeling defeated right now. She has some warm chicken broth for me, and she asks me how I'm doing. I told her I was starting to fall asleep out there. Right away she looks at me, and realizes what's going on. "No, you're not falling asleep. You're hypothermic. You're trying to pass out." We go back to the tent, and she does the best she can to warm me up. I drink hot coffee as she pours hot water on my hands and feet and puts a blanket over my shoulders.

Jess did awesome as my pit crew. I prepared her going into it and told her everything she needed to do for me during the race. She would need to help me organize my gear and help me figure out when I need to change in and out of gear. Help keep me fueled between laps. Help make sure I drink water so I stay hydrated and keep from cramping up during the race. I also told her there may be a time, maybe around 2:00 a.m., where my spirits may be really down and I may want to quit. It would be up to her to bring me out of it. Weeks before the race, I told her about the possibility of my spirit breaking in the night. I didn't think it was true, though. I just figured since I've done this race twice now, I'm a two-time World's Toughest Mudder already, so I know what this takes. This is 12 hours of physical strength, followed by 12 hours of mental strength. This is just about how much can you take and keep going. There's nothing that this course is going to throw at me that I can't take. I believed that with all of my heart. Knowing that made this moment so much harder.

The cold that Mother Nature threw us was a game changer. It was over ten hours of below freezing temperatures. There was frost on the ground. There was frost on the tents. There was frost on everything in sight. There were hardly any headlamps on the course because so many people had dropped out of the race by now. They actually closed down five obstacles because they were covered in sheets of ice. At this point, I was past the point of wanting to quit and I just felt broken. I felt like there was just nothing left for me to give. I felt like a failure. I felt defeated. I was in a dark place.

I know Jess had never seen me in that place before. It's probably a safe bet to say no one's ever seen me in that place before. It was pretty bad. Even though she'd never seen me there before, she came ready. She enlisted an army of my clients, my friends, and my family for this very moment. She had them write letters for me so I could open them when I needed encouragement. The notes were full of reminders about how inspiring they think I am, what I'm made of, what I'm capable of, and that they believe in me. There was even a note from our dog, Walter, who was sad he couldn't be there but was rooting for me at home. She had updated posts on Facebook, and every time someone made a comment, she relayed those inspiring words to me. Those words were like spinach to me, and they gave me energy. I was still really struggling, but that gave me enough energy to help push me through and get back on the course.

Not only was I able to get back on the course, but I completed two more laps. I was able to make it to 40 miles, which was my goal. Forty miles at 40 years old. I know I would not have made it to my goal if Jess had not helped me through that tough time during the race. It taught me a valuable lesson. I do these obstacle races because I feel like they make me stronger as a person. After I go through these obstacles and take on these challenging courses, it translates over to my life. Then whenever I face challenges and obstacles in life, I feel like I'm able to handle them better. We all face obstacles all the time. When we come up against an obstacle, we have two choices: either we can overcome the obstacle or the obstacle can overcome us. The lesson I learned from this race was that the bigger the obstacle or the challenge we face, the more important it is that we have a strong pit crew. Jess can't take the pain away for me. She can't go through the course for me, but she can be there with me and ease my suffering. She can push me through that struggle to help me get to my best so I can reach my goals.

Ask yourself who your pit crew is. How strong is your pit crew? When you face obstacles in life are they enabling you to take the easy way out and quit, or are they pushing you through your struggle so you can reach your goals?

Action Step: Let's take a look at your pit crew

Who is your pit crew?

_____

_____

_____

How strong is your pit crew?

_____

_____

_____

Nutrition: Pre- and Post-Workout Tips

The nutrition tips I offer in this week's nutrition section are just that, tips. I am not a dietician or a nutritionist. These are just things that I have learned over the last 15 years in fitness to work best for myself and my clients. Keep in mind that every body is different, and what works best for me or my clients may not be what works best for you. In order to really learn what works best for you pre-workout and post-workout may take a little trial and error to figure out.

Pre-Workout Snack/Meal:

Your goal for your pre-workout snack or meal needs to be centered around two things: energy and performance. You have to find the right window of time between your last meal or your pre-workout snack and your workout. You need to have long enough so that your food can be digested and not make you nauseated, but not so long that you run out of fuel before the workout is over. I have found that about 60–90 minutes is usually about right for a meal, and usually 45–60 minutes is good for a lighter snack. You want to make sure your meal or snack includes both protein and carbs. There are many pre-workout supplements out there that people love, but I would tread lightly. Many will make you jittery and have a negative effect on your performance. If it is too sugary, it may cause you to have energy at first, but then you may crash in the middle of your workout. I have found that good sleep, hydration, and nutrition tend to work better for me.

Post-Workout Snack/Meal:

Your goal for your post-workout snack or meal should be about recovery and refueling. First, you want to be rehydrating yourself both during and after your workout. The more water you lose during your workout (sweat), the more you need to rehydrate. Within 30 minutes of a resistance training workout, I like to have a recovery meal or recovery shake. This meal has a 2:1 ratio of carbs to protein and usually 200–300 calories. I have found that having this recovery meal will greatly decrease your body's recovery time after a workout. If you are someone who is always really sore after your workouts, I would first look at your nutrition. A recovery meal or shake after your workouts may make a big difference. Within 90 minutes of your workout, I would then have a full meal.

Action Steps: What works best for you

When it comes to your pre- and post-workout eating routine, it takes being observant to really learn what works best for you. For the next few days, take notes about the following things:

What did you eat before your workout? How long was it before your workout?

_____

_____

_____

How did you feel during the workout?

_____

_____

_____

What did you eat after the workout? How soon was it after your workout?

_____

_____

_____

How did you feel after your workout? How fast did you bounce back? Were you sore the next day? If so, how sore?

_____

_____

_____

Training: What Are You Made Of?

Sometimes you just need a change of pace with your workouts. Maybe they get boring or you lose a little motivation to go do them. After hosting a Saturday bootcamp for many years, I decided to throw a curveball at everyone and add a new challenge. That is how I got the idea for my Sunday bootcamps called "What Are You Made Of?"

About once a month, I put on one of these Sunday bootcamps, which are designed to push my attendees a little harder than my Saturday bootcamp does. Hard workouts will help you increase your mental strength just as much as your physical strength, and it will translate to your job, your family, and your fitness. We are forced to face obstacles and challenges every day. When obstacles show up in our lives, we have two choices . . . we can overcome the obstacle or we can let the obstacle overcome us. Every time you choose to dig a little deeper and push through hard challenges, you grow stronger. These workouts help you find out what you are made of.

You can find a list and description of our past "What Are You Made Of?" workouts here:

https://overlandparkfitness.com/finish-strong/

Finish Strong

The mental strength and toughness that you can gain from a hard workout is another benefit of exercise that we take for granted. Another way you can get this benefit is simply by finishing your workout strong. When we get to the end of a workout, we are usually pretty spent, both physically and mentally. Being able to dig deep and find enough energy to finish as strong as you started is a very good habit to create in yourself. In no time, you will start to see that "Finish Strong" habits carry over into all other areas of your life.

I like to give my clients workout finishers at the very end of their workouts from time to time, to help them build this habit. I call these workout finishers Overtime Circuits.

You can find a list and description of some of my Overtime Circuits here:

https://overlandparkfitness.com/finish-strong/

Action Steps: Finish strong with workout finishers

How can adding in a few harder workouts to your routine help you?

_____

_____

_____

Go to the links above to check out my "What Are You Made Of?" workouts and Overtime Circuits.

Weekly Fitness Evaluation Form

Now, it is time to give yourself a grade for the week. By doing this weekly self-evaluation and asking yourself the questions on this sheet, you will learn how to keep yourself accountable to your fitness plan. Every week you will learn more from doing this evaluation, and before long your fitness plan will become a top priority in your life.

Here is how this works: Answer the questions below, and then grade yourself for the week. If you give yourself an A+, awesome! All you have to do is just keep it up. If you don't give yourself an A+, ask yourself what went wrong. What obstacles got in your way? How can you overcome these obstacles in the future? These questions will help you when setting yourself up for next week's success.

First, let's start with what you did well . . .

Name three things you are proud of after this week:

1._____

2._____

3._____

Mindset

How was your energy this week? If it was low, did you get enough sleep? Did you drink enough water? What other factors could've affected your energy?

_____

_____

_____

How did you feel during your workouts this week? (Ex: strong or weak, athletic or uncoordinated, tired or energetic)

_____

_____

_____

How was your motivation this week? Was it easy to get your workouts in or challenging? Was it easy to stick to the healthy guidelines or challenging?

_____

_____

_____

What grade do you give your mindset for this week? ___

Nutrition

Did you throw out the temptations and replace them with healthier options?

_____

_____

_____

Did you follow a meal plan? Did you get all your meals in? Did you drink enough water?

_____

_____

_____

Did you have any treats or cheats? If yes, what were your cheat meals? Were they intentional or unplanned?

_____

_____

_____

What grade do you give your nutrition this week? ___

Training

Did you get all of your workouts in this week (resistance training and cardio training)? If your answer is no, which workouts did you miss/skip? Why didn't you get them in?

_____

_____

_____

Did you need to make modifications to any exercises this week? If yes, which exercises, and why/how did you modify them?

_____

_____

_____

What grade do you give your workouts this week? ___

You will use your answers to the questions in this evaluation in the next section, "Set Yourself Up for Success."

Set Yourself Up for Success
for Next Week

Now, it's time to set yourself up for success for the upcoming week. Your fitness goals are no different than anything else you want to accomplish in life. If you don't have a plan, then you might as well plan to fail. The action steps in this form are designed to help you reach your goals in the week ahead.

The first thing we're going to do is overcome the biggest excuse that we always make: "I don't have time." We love this excuse, and it is the easiest one to use.

Make Time

We are going to overcome this excuse right now by making time. The way you make time is scheduling your workouts.

Step 1: Go to your online training program and click on your calendar. I have scheduled your workouts out for the week, but you have the ability to drag and move them to whatever day you'd like. (Not doing one of my online training programs? No problem. You can use your phone calendar or your desk calendar, and just move your workouts around any conflicts.)

Step 2: Identify any conflicts that could affect your workouts getting completed. Look at your work schedule this week. Do you have to travel this week? Are there any meetings or events you need to be at that could be overlapping a scheduled workout? Now look at your family calendar. What family stuff is going on this week? Do you have a family event or activity going on this week? Do you have a date with a significant other? Do your kids have activities or events this week? What conflicts present themselves?

Step 3: Drag and move your workouts around any conflicts that you face this week. (It is ok to do resistance training workouts on consecutive days if you have to in order to get them in. Ideally, you want to have a rest day between them when possible. It is also ok to do a resistance training workout and a cardio workout on the same day.)

Step 4: Plan out what time of day you will be doing each workout. (In the morning before work, during lunch, after work, on your day off. . .)

Plan Out Your Meals

What I have found to be the most successful way of keeping myself honest to a healthy eating plan throughout the week is meal prepping at the beginning of the week. You must plan out what you're going to eat throughout the week, and prepare it before the week starts. This helps set you up for success. So for example, if I know that every day for breakfast (or for one of my early morning snacks) I'm going to have two hard-boiled eggs and a banana, then on Sunday I'll purchase it, prepare it, and get it ready for the entire week. Meal prepping like this at the beginning of the week, for as many meals and snacks as you can, will help you succeed.

Step 1: In the first chart below, write out everything you plan to eat for your meals and snacks for the upcoming week. (If you are like me and eat the same thing for breakfast every day and repeat snacks often, this will not take very long.) As you fill this out for the week, be sure to write down any planned dinners out, work-related lunches or other meals, events, happy hours, etc.

Step 2: Look over the meals and snacks you planned out for the week and use the second chart to create your grocery list.

Step 3: Get your groceries for the week.

Step 4: Cook/prepare all of your meals for the week.

Meals / Snacks

	Breakfast	AM Snack (optional)	Lunch	PM Snack (optional)	Dinner
Monday					
Tuesday					
Wednesday					
Thursday					
Friday					
Saturday					
Sunday					

Grocery List
1.
2.
3.
4.
5.
6.
7.
8.
9.
10.

Bonus Material

A Letter to the New Me

What do I want to accomplish in the next three months?

_____

_____

_____

A goal without a plan is not a goal . . . it is a wish. I understand that in order to accomplish my goals I need to have a plan of attack that best fits me and my life.

My plan to reach my fitness goals:

My plan for my workouts (when, where, how often, how long, who with...any other details):

_____

_____

_____

My intentions for my nutrition (What will I eat, what will I not eat. Any other important details.):

_____

_____

_____

Other intentions:

_____

_____

_____

Sticking to the plan:

You can have the best game plan in the world to help you reach your goals, but if you don't hold yourself accountable to it, it will not work. In order to succeed, you need to consistently hold yourself accountable to your plan.

How will I keep myself accountable and consistent to my plan?

_____

_____

_____

Getting Back Up:

Failing is inevitable. I know I will fail from time to time, but failing does not define me nor does it stop me from reaching my goals. What defines me is how I respond to failing.

How will I get myself back on track if I fail?

_____

_____

_____

Start Your Day Right

How you start your day can affect the rest of your day. You can begin your day in a good mood by doing some easy things in the morning that will have you leaving your house expecting to have a wonderful day.

Step 1: Smile

Begin every day with a smile. Even if it is for no apparent reason. Despite whatever happened the day before, it is a new day. You have a fresh start, and today you can choose to be in a good mood. Start with a ten-second smile. It will make you feel better and will make everyone around you feel better. A smile will set a good tone for the rest of the day.

Step 2: Take a Breath

Paying attention to your breathing is one of the fastest ways to become calm and centered. For at least a little, while do not think about your problems or the tasks you have ahead of you. Just take some deep long breaths in through your nose and out through your mouth. This will help you wake up calm and refreshed.

Step 3: Be Grateful

Begin your morning with an attitude of gratitude.

We can complain because rose bushes have thorns, or we can rejoice because thorn bushes have roses.
~Abraham Lincoln

Attitude is everything! Take some time to think of three to five things that you are grateful for right now.

Action Steps: Everyday do something that makes you happy!

If you don't already, begin to incorporate the above tasks in your morning routine. What are some things you love doing that you could do more of in the morning? (Ex: Listening to music, reading, singing, meditation, yoga)

_____

_____

_____

Starting your day with happiness can fill your whole day with happiness.
Happiness is not something you postpone for the future; it is something you design for the present.
~ Jim Rohn

Weekly Fitness Evaluation Form

Now, it is time to give yourself a grade for the week. By doing this weekly self-evaluation and asking yourself the questions on this sheet, you will learn how to keep yourself accountable to your fitness plan. Every week you will learn more from doing this evaluation, and before long your fitness plan will become a top priority in your life.

Here is how this works: Answer the questions below, and then grade yourself for the week. If you give yourself an A+, awesome! All you have to do is just keep it up. If you don't give yourself an A+, ask yourself what went wrong. What obstacles got in your way? How can you overcome these obstacles in the future? These questions will help you when setting yourself up for next week's success.

First, let's start with what you did well . . .

Name three things you are proud of after this week:

1._____

2._____

3._____

Mindset

How was your energy this week? If it was low, did you get enough sleep? Did you drink enough water? What other factors could've affected your energy?

_____

_____

_____

How did you feel during your workouts this week? (Ex: strong or weak, athletic or uncoordinated, tired or energetic)

_____

_____

_____

How was your motivation this week? Was it easy to get your workouts in or challenging? Was it easy to stick to the healthy guidelines or challenging?

_____

_____

_____

What grade do you give your mindset for this week? ___

Nutrition

Did you throw out the temptations and replace them with healthier options?

_____

_____

_____

Did you follow a meal plan? Did you get all your meals in? Did you drink enough water?

_____

_____

_____

Did you have any treats or cheats? If yes, what were your cheat meals? Were they intentional or unplanned?

_____

_____

_____

What grade do you give your nutrition this week? ___

Training

Did you get all of your workouts in this week (resistance training and cardio training)? If your answer is no, which workouts did you miss/skip? Why didn't you get them in?

_____

_____

_____

Did you need to make modifications to any exercises this week? If yes, which exercises, and why/how did you modify them?

_____

_____

_____

What grade do you give your workouts this week? ___

You will use your answers to the questions in this evaluation in the next section, "Set Yourself Up for Success."

Set Yourself Up For Success

Now, it's time to set yourself up for success for the upcoming week. Your fitness goals are no different than anything else you want to accomplish in life. If you don't have a plan, then you might as well plan to fail. The action steps in this form are designed to help you reach your goals in the week ahead.

The first thing we're going to do is overcome the biggest excuse that we always make: "I don't have time." We love this excuse, and it is the easiest one to use.

Make Time

We are going to overcome this excuse right now by making time. The way you make time is scheduling your workouts.

Step 1: Go to your online training program and click on your calendar. I have scheduled your workouts out for the week, but you have the ability to drag and move them to whatever day you'd like. (Not doing one of my online training programs? No problem. You can use your phone calendar or your desk calendar, and just move your workouts around any conflicts.)

Step 2: Identify any conflicts that could affect your workouts getting completed. Look at your work schedule this week. Do you have to travel this week? Are there any meetings or events you need to be at that could be overlapping a scheduled workout? Now look at your family calendar. What family stuff is going on this week? Do you have a family event or activity going on this week? Do you have a date with a significant other? Do your kids have activities or events this week? What conflicts present themselves?

Step 3: Drag and move your workouts around any conflicts that you face this week. (It is ok to do resistance training workouts on consecutive days if you have to in order to get them in. Ideally, you want to have a rest day between them when possible. It is also ok to do a resistance training workout and a cardio workout on the same day.)

Step 4: Plan out what time of day you will be doing each workout. (In the morning before work, during lunch, after work, on your day off...)

Plan Out Your Meals

What I have found to be the most successful way of keeping myself honest to a healthy eating plan throughout the week is meal prepping at the beginning of the week. You must plan out what you're going to eat throughout the week, and prepare it before the week starts. This helps set you up for success. So for example, if I know that every day for breakfast (or for one of my early morning snacks) I'm going to have two hard-boiled eggs and a banana, then on Sunday I'll purchase it, prepare it, and get it ready for the entire week. Meal prepping like this at the beginning of the week, for as many meals and snacks as you can, will help you succeed.

Step 1: In the first chart below, write out everything you plan to eat for your meals and snacks for the upcoming week. (If you are like me and eat the same thing for breakfast every day and repeat snacks often, this will not take very long.) As you fill this out for the week, be sure to write down any planned dinners out, work-related lunches or other meals, events, happy hours, etc.

Step 2: Look over the meals and snacks you planned out for the week and use the second chart to create your grocery list.

Step 3: Get your groceries for the week.

Step 4: Cook/prepare all of your meals for the week.

Meals / Snacks					
	Breakfast	AM Snack (optional)	Lunch	PM Snack (optional)	Dinner
Monday					
Tuesday					
Wednesday					
Thursday					
Friday					
Saturday					
Sunday					

Grocery List
1.
2.
3.
4.
5.
6.
7.
8.
9.
10.

About the Author

Chad Austin has been a leader in the fitness industry since 2003. He has experience as an athlete, coach, student, teacher, client, and trainer. He has been a full-time personal trainer since 2006. Chad Austin is the owner of Priority Fitness in Overland Park, Kansas. Priority Fitness was named after his best-selling book, *Make Fitness A Priority: How to Win the Fight Against Your Excuses*. Chad is the co-founder of the health and fitness meet-up group, Make Fitness A Priority, a group for all fitness levels lead by fitness professionals. He was voted a Top 10 personal trainer in Kansas City by Thumbtack Professionals in 2015 and 2016, and was featured in KC Fitness Magazine as one of the Faces Shaping KC in 2013 and 2014.

Chad's definition of fitness is to constantly strive to be better than you were the day before, the week before, and the month before in regard to your physical and mental health. He believes that in fitness anything is possible when you take the right progressions to achieve your goal.

Made in the
USA
Columbia, SC